DIABETIC RENAL DIET COOKBOOK FOR SENIORS

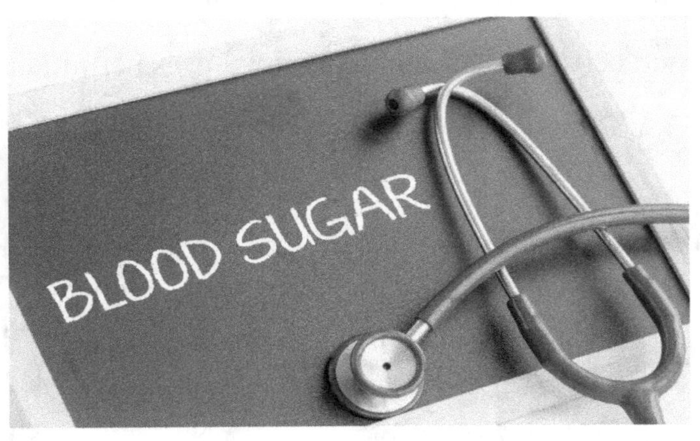

Nutritious Recipes for Health and Well-being

Jessica G farmer

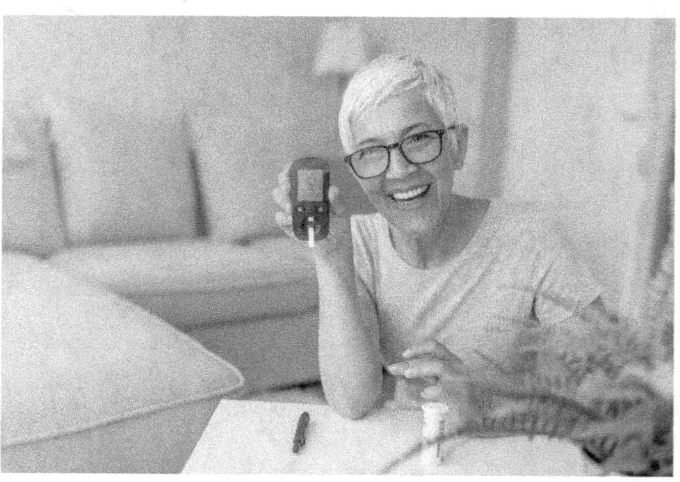

Table of contents

INTRODUCTION

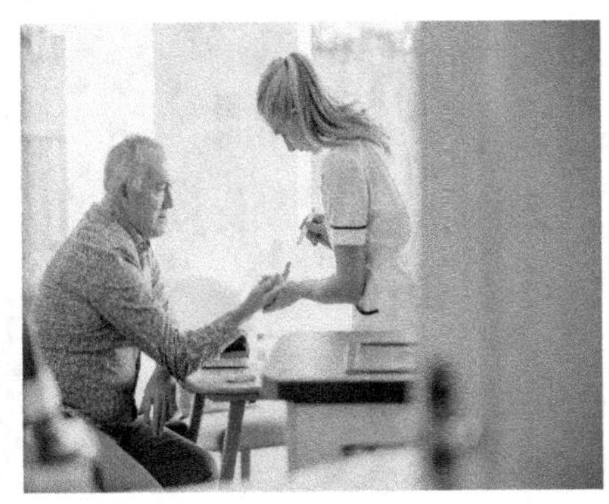 Wilson was a young-at-heart senior who enjoyed being active and had always taken pleasure in leading a healthy lifestyle. He delighted in gardening, taking long strolls in the park, and cooking delectable dinners for his family. But when he was told he had kidney problems and diabetes, his life took an unexpected turn.

Wilson realized he needed to drastically alter his diet to adequately manage his health as he struggled with the realities of his situation. His physician advised him to follow a diabetic renal diet, a particular eating regimen that would promote the health of his kidneys while also assisting in the management of his blood sugar levels. Wilson set out on a quest to learn more about this eating regimen because he was determined to recover his vigour.

Wilson started doing in-depth studies due to his inquisitive personality and hunger for information. To learn more about the diabetic renal diet, he researched numerous internet forums, medical websites, and nutritionists. Although he discovered several resources, he was looking for something more usable and easily accessible—something that could lead him step by step.

One day, Wilson was perusing his neighbourhood bookshop when he came upon a cookbook for seniors with diabetes and kidney disease. The colourful pictures of tasty food on the cover drew his attention. He snatched it up out of curiosity and began leafing through the pages. A wealth of knowledge, simple-to-follow recipes, and practical advice for those managing diabetes and kidney problems were all included in the book.

Wilson immediately bought the cookbook after his discovery and went home. He discovered as he looked over its contents that it was a gold mine of culinary ideas. The cookbook gave information on the nutritional advantages of different foods and cooking methods in addition to offering complete meal plans.

Wilson's acquired cookbook quickly established itself as his go-to cooking partner. Lean proteins, whole grains, a variety of fresh vegetables, fruits, and other kidney-friendly components were among the elements he started experimenting with in his dishes. He learned about a variety of herbs and spices from the cookbook that enhanced the taste of his food without sacrificing its nutritional value.

Wilson's self-assurance in the kitchen rose week by week. He loved the smell of soups boiling, the sizzle of stir-fried veggies, and the pleasure of preparing scrumptious but wholesome meals. He found a world of sensations he had never had before, and it gave him hope that despite his health issues, he could still have a satisfying diet.

Wilson's commitment to the diabetic renal diet and his newly discovered culinary abilities were noted. The delicious meals he cooked were admired by his family and friends, who were unaware that they had been thoughtfully designed to promote his health. They were inspired by his fortitude and will to survive while still appreciating the basic joys of eating.

Wilson's health started to become better over time. His blood sugar levels returned to normal, and his kidney function seemed to be improving. He was thankful for the adventure he had done and felt more powerful and energised. The diabetic renal diet had evolved into more than a way for him to control his health; it had evolved into a way for him to change and gain power.

Wilson was overcome with thankfulness for the diabetic renal diet cookbook, which had led him on his road to recovery as he thought back on his experience. It had been his devoted travel partner, encouraging him at every turn. Inspired by his experience, he decided to reach out to others who may be going through similar difficulties with his tale and the priceless resource that had made a huge impact on his life.

Wilson went out to promote the value of an appropriate diet in the treatment of diabetes and kidney problems with a newfound sense of purpose. He set out to encourage and enable other older citizens to take charge of their health and embrace the transformational power of food, armed with his cookbook and the information he had learnt.

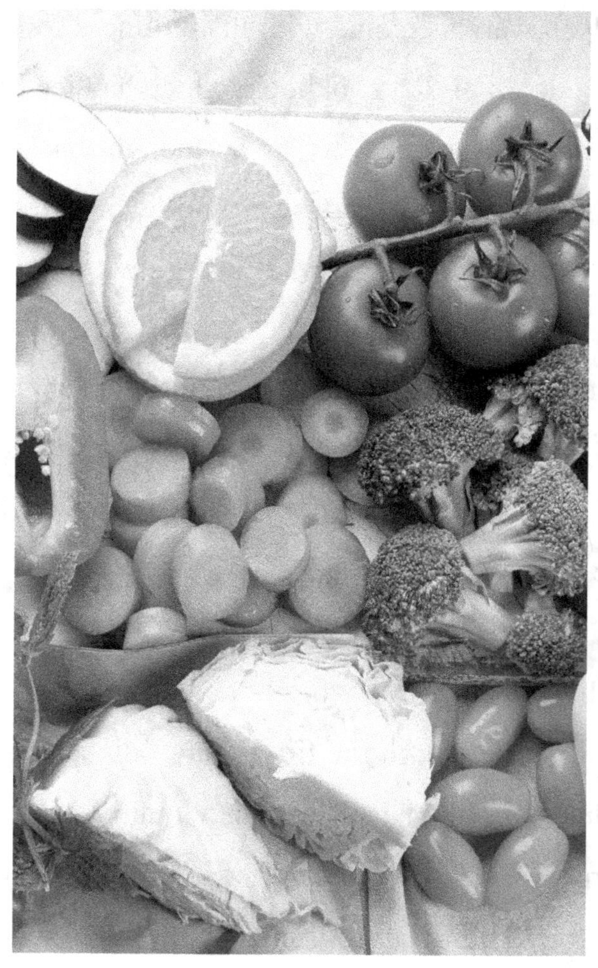

CHAPTER 1 BREAKFAST RECIPES

Vegetable Omelette

Ingredients

- 4 eggs
- 1/4 cup milk
- Salt and pepper to taste
- 1 tablespoon butter or oil
- 1/2 onion, chopped
- 1 bell pepper, diced
- 1 small zucchini, diced
- 1 cup sliced mushrooms
- 1 cup baby spinach
- 1/2 cup shredded cheese (cheddar, mozzarella, or your choice)

Instructions

1. In a bowl, whisk the eggs and milk together. Season with salt and pepper to taste. Set aside. Heat the butter or oil in a non-stick skillet over medium heat. Add the chopped onion, bell pepper, zucchini, and mushrooms to the skillet. Sauté for about 5 minutes or until the vegetables are tender. Add the baby spinach to the skillet and cook until wilted.

2. Remove the vegetables from the skillet and set aside. Wipe the skillet clean with a paper towel and return it to the stove over medium heat.

3. Add a little more butter or oil to the skillet, making sure to coat the bottom.

4. Pour the egg mixture into the skillet, tilting the pan to spread the eggs evenly.

5. Cook the omelette for a few minutes until the edges start to set. Sprinkle the sautéed vegetables evenly over one-half of the omelette.

6. Sprinkle the shredded cheese over the vegetables. Using a spatula, carefully fold the other half of the omelette over the filling, creating a half-moon shape.

7. Cook for another minute or until the cheese has melted and the omelette is cooked through. Carefully transfer the omelette to a plate and cut it into wedges. Serve hot and enjoy!

Greek Yogurt Parfait

Ingredients

- 2 cups Greek yogurt
- 1 cup granola
- 1 cup mixed berries (such as strawberries, blueberries, and raspberries)
- 2 tablespoons honey
- 1 teaspoon vanilla extract
- Fresh mint leaves (for garnish, optional)

Instructions

1. In a bowl, blend the Greek yoghurt, honey, and vanilla concentrate until very much consolidated. This will be the yoghurt layer of your parfait.

2. Take serving glasses or bowls and begin layering the fixings. Start with a spoonful of the Greek yoghurt blend as the base layer.

3. Add a layer of granola on top of the yoghurt. You can pick your number one granola or make your own.

4. Then, add a layer of blended berries on top of the granola. Go ahead and utilize various berries or simply stick to one kind.

5. Rehash the layers with one more spoonful of Greek yoghurt blend, trailed by granola, and afterwards blended

berries. Keep layering until the glasses or bowls are filled.

6. Polish off the parfait with a bit of the Greek yoghurt combination on the exceptional top layer.

7. Whenever wanted, decorate with a couple of new mint leaves for added newness and show.

8. Serve the Greek Yogurt Parfait right away and appreciate it!

Quinoa Breakfast Bowl

Ingredients

- 1 cup quinoa
- 2 cups water
- 1 cup almond milk (or any other plant-based milk)
- 1 tablespoon maple syrup (or honey)
- 1 teaspoon vanilla extract
- 1/2 teaspoon ground cinnamon

- Pinch of salt

- Fresh berries (such as strawberries, blueberries, or raspberries)

- Sliced banana

- Chopped nuts (such as almonds, walnuts, or pecans)

- Unsweetened shredded coconut

- Chia seeds

Instructions

1. Wash the quinoa under chilly water to eliminate any harsh buildup. In a pan, join the quinoa and water. Heat to the point of boiling, then, at that point, lessen the intensity to low, cover, and stew for around 15 minutes or until the quinoa is delicate and the water is ingested.

2. In a different little pot, heat the almond milk over medium-low intensity. Mix in the maple syrup, vanilla concentrate,

cinnamon, and a spot of salt. Heat the combination for a couple of moments until warmed through and very much joined.

3. Once the quinoa is cooked, cushion it with a fork. Pour the warm almond milk combination over the cooked quinoa and mix tenderly to join.

4. Partition the quinoa combination into serving bowls. Top each bowl with new berries, cut bananas, cleaved nuts, destroyed coconut, and a sprinkle of chia seeds.

5. Serve the quinoa breakfast bowls warm and Appreciative.

Whole Grain Toast with Avocado and Egg

Ingredients:

- 2 slices of whole grain bread

- 1 ripe avocado

- 2 eggs

- Salt and pepper to taste

- Optional toppings: red pepper flakes, chia seeds, or fresh herbs

Instructions

1. Toast the bread: Spot the cuts of entire grain bread in a toaster oven or toaster and toast them until they are brilliant brown and firm.

2. Set up the avocado: Cut the ready avocado down the middle, eliminate the pit, and scoop out the tissue into a little bowl. Squash the avocado with a fork until it arrives at your ideal consistency. Add salt and pepper to taste and blend well.

3. Cook the eggs: Intensity a non-stick skillet over medium intensity. Break the eggs into the skillet, they are not

excessively near one another to guarantee that they. Sprinkle a spot of salt and pepper over the eggs. Cook the eggs to your favoured degree of doneness, for example, just right or done on both sides.

4. Collect the toast: Take the toasted bread cuts and spread the crushed avocado equally over each cut.

5. Add the eggs: Cautiously put one cooked egg on top of every avocado-shrouded cut of bread.

6. Season and topping: Sprinkle some extra salt and pepper over the eggs. Whenever wanted, add discretionary garnishes like red pepper pieces, chia seeds, or new spices for additional flavour and surface.

7. Serve and appreciate: Spot the collected entire grain toast with avocado and egg on a plate and serve quickly while the eggs are still warm.

Cottage Cheese with Fresh Fruit

Ingredients:

- 1 cup cottage cheese
- Assorted fresh fruits (such as berries, sliced peaches, sliced bananas, diced mango, etc.)
- 1 tablespoon honey (optional)
- 2 tablespoons chopped nuts (optional, for garnish)

Instructions

1. Begin by setting up the new natural products. Wash them completely under running water and wipe them off. Cut or dice the natural products as wanted and saved them.

2. Take a serving bowl or individual dishes for individual servings. Spoon the curds into the bowl(s) and spread it uniformly.

3. Orchestrate the different new organic products on top of the curds. You can be inventive and make an outwardly engaging game plan by utilizing various tones and surfaces of natural products.

4. If you lean toward a dash of pleasantness, sprinkle honey over the curds and natural products. The honey will upgrade the flavours and add characteristic pleasantness.

5. Sprinkle hacked nuts on top of the curds and natural products for added crunch and flavour. You can utilize almonds, pecans, walnuts, or some other nuts of your decision.

6. When the curds with the new organic product are ready, it is prepared to serve. Appreciate it as an invigorating breakfast, a light bite, or a solid pastry.

Spinach and Mushroom Scramble

Ingredients:

- 4 large eggs
- 1 cup spinach leaves, washed and chopped
- 1 cup mushrooms, sliced
- 1/2 onion, diced
- 2 cloves of garlic, minced
- 2 tablespoons olive oil
- Salt and pepper to taste
- Optional toppings: grated cheese, chopped fresh herbs (such as parsley or chives)

Instructions

1. Heat one tablespoon of olive oil in a huge non-stick skillet over medium intensity.

2. Add the diced onion and minced garlic to the skillet and sauté until the onion becomes clear and fragrant.

3. Add the cut mushrooms to the skillet and cook until they begin to mellow and deliver their dampness, around 5 minutes.

4. Mix in the slashed spinach and cook for an extra 2-3 minutes until the spinach shrivels.

5. In the interim, break the eggs into a bowl and whisk them together until very much consolidated. Season with salt and pepper.

6. Push the vegetables aside from the skillet and empty the whisked eggs into the vacant space.

7. Permit the eggs to cook for a couple of moments until they begin to set around the edges.

8. Delicately scramble the eggs with a spatula, consolidating the vegetables as you go.

9. Proceed to cook and mix until the eggs are completely cooked yet at the same time soggy.

10. Eliminate the skillet from intensity and shower the excess tablespoon of olive oil over the scramble. Throw everything together to guarantee even dispersion of flavours.

11. Taste and change the flavouring if necessary.

12. Serve the Spinach and Mushroom Scramble hot with your #1 garnishes like ground cheddar or slashed new spices.

Sweet Potato Breakfast Hash

Ingredients:

- 2 medium sweet potatoes, peeled and diced
- 1 red bell pepper, diced
- 1 small red onion, diced
- 2 cloves of garlic, minced
- 4 slices of bacon, chopped
- 4 eggs
- 2 tablespoons olive oil
- 1 teaspoon paprika
- 1/2 teaspoon cumin
- Salt and pepper to taste
- Fresh parsley, chopped (for garnish)

Instructions

1. Heat an enormous skillet over medium intensity and add the hacked bacon. Cook until fresh, then, at that point, eliminate from the skillet and put away. Leave the bacon oil in the skillet.

2. In a similar skillet with the bacon oil, add the olive oil and intensity over

medium-high intensity. Add the diced yams and cook for around 5 minutes, blending once in a while, until they begin to relax.

3. Add the diced red chime pepper and red onion to the skillet and cook for an additional 5 minutes, or until the vegetables are delicate.

4. Mix in the minced garlic, paprika, cumin, salt, and pepper. Cook for an extra 1-2 minutes, until the flavours are fragrant.

5. Make four little wells in the yam blend and break an egg into each well. Lessen the intensity to medium-low, cover the skillet, and cook for around 5-7 minutes, or until the eggs are cooked to your ideal doneness.

6. Sprinkle the cooked bacon over the hash and embellishment with new parsley.

7. Serve the Yam Breakfast Hash hot, straightforwardly from the skillet. You can appreciate it with no guarantees or with a side of toast or a new natural product.

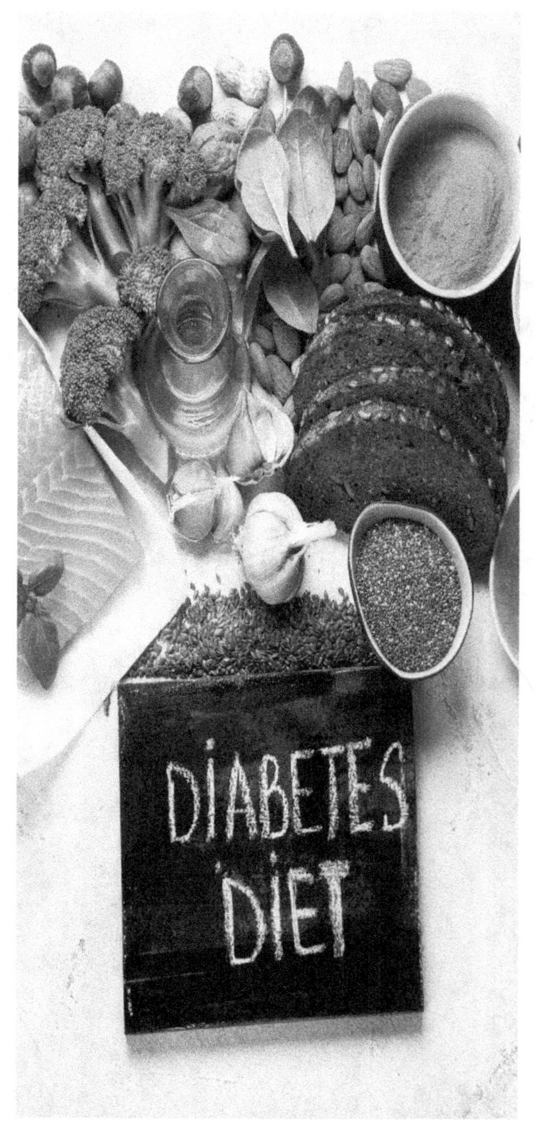
DIABETES
DIET

CHAPTER 2 :LUNCH RECIPES

Grilled Chicken Salad

Ingredients:

- 2 boneless, skinless chicken breasts
- Salt and pepper, to taste
- 2 tablespoons olive oil
- 8 cups mixed salad greens
- 1 cup cherry tomatoes, halved
- 1 cucumber, sliced
- 1 red bell pepper, sliced
- 1/4 red onion, thinly sliced
- 1/2 cup crumbled feta cheese
- 1/4 cup sliced black olives
- 1/4 cup chopped fresh basil
- For the dressing:
- 1/4 cup olive oil
- 2 tablespoons lemon juice

- 1 clove garlic, minced
- 1 teaspoon Dijon mustard
- Salt and pepper, to taste

Instructions

1. Preheat your barbecue to medium-high intensity.

2. Season the chicken bosoms with salt and pepper on the two sides. Shower them with olive oil, they are equally covered to ensure they.

3. Put the chicken bosoms on the preheated barbecue and cook for around 6-8 minutes for every side, or until the inward temperature comes to 165°F (74°C). Eliminate them from the barbecue and let them rest for a couple of moments before cutting.

4. While the chicken is resting, set up the serving of mixed greens. In an enormous bowl, join the blended plate of mixed

greens, cherry tomatoes, cucumber, red ringer pepper, red onion, feta cheddar, and dark olives.

5. In a little bowl, whisk together the additional virgin olive oil, lemon juice, Dijon mustard, minced garlic, salt, and pepper to make the dressing.

6. Cut the barbecued chicken bosoms into flimsy strips.

7. Add the cut chicken to the plate of mixed greens and sprinkle the dressing over the top. Throw everything together until it is all1p1p1 around covered.

8. Serve the barbecued chicken plate of mixed greens right away, embellished with new spices whenever wanted

Baked Salmon with Steamed Vegetables

Ingredients:

- 4 salmon fillets

- 1 lemon, sliced

- 2 tablespoons olive oil

- Salt and pepper to taste

- 1 teaspoon garlic powder

- 1 teaspoon dried dill (optional)

- 4 cups mixed vegetables (such as broccoli, carrots, and cauliflower)

Instructions

1. Preheat your broiler to 400°F (200°C). Line a baking sheet with material paper or aluminium foil.

2. Put the salmon filets on the pre-arranged baking sheet. Shower them with olive oil and crush the juice from half of the lemon over the filets. Season with salt, pepper, garlic powder, and dried dill. Put a couple of lemon cuts on top of each filet.

3. Heat the salmon in the preheated stove for around 12-15 minutes, or until the fish drops effectively with a fork and is cooked to your ideal degree of doneness.

4. While the salmon is heating up, set up the steamed vegetables. Fill a pot with around 1 inch of water and heat it to the point of boiling. Place a liner bin or colander over the bubbling water, ensuring it doesn't contact the water.

5. Add the blended vegetables to the liner container. Cover the pot with a top and steam the vegetables for around 5-7 minutes, or until they are delicate yet still marginally fresh.

6. When the salmon and vegetables are cooked, eliminate them from the broiler and liner bin, individually.

7. Serve the prepared salmon on a plate close by the steamed vegetables. Crush the excess lemon juice over the salmon

and vegetables for additional newness. You can decorate with new dill, whenever wanted.

Turkey Lettuce Wraps

Ingredients:

- 1 pound ground turkey
- 2 tablespoons vegetable oil
- 3 cloves garlic, minced
- 1 small onion, finely chopped
- 1 red bell pepper, finely chopped
- 1 carrot, grated
- 2 tablespoons soy sauce
- 1 tablespoon hoisin sauce
- 1 teaspoon sesame oil
- 1 teaspoon ginger, grated
- Salt and pepper to taste
- 1 head lettuce (such as iceberg or butter lettuce), leaves separated and washed

- Optional toppings: chopped green onions, chopped peanuts, cilantro leaves

Instructions

1. Heat the vegetable oil in an enormous skillet or wok over medium-high intensity.
2. Add the garlic, onion, and ringer pepper to the skillet and sauté until the vegetables are delicate.
3. Add the ground turkey to the skillet and cook, separating it with a spoon, until it is sautéed and cooked through.
4. Mix in the ground carrot, soy sauce, hoisin sauce, sesame oil, and ginger. Cook for an extra 2-3 minutes to permit the flavours to merge.
5. Season with salt and pepper to taste.
6. Eliminate the skillet from the intensity and let the combination cool marginally.

7. Orchestrate the lettuce leaves on a serving platter.

8. Spoon the turkey combination onto every lettuce leaf, isolating it equally.

9. Discretionary: Sprinkle with cleaved green onions, slashed peanuts, and cilantro leaves for added flavour and trimming.

10. Serve right away and partake in the Turkey Lettuce Wraps as a light and solid starter or principal course.

Quinoa and Vegetable Stir-Fry

Ingredients:

- 1 cup quinoa
- 2 cups water
- 2 tablespoons vegetable oil
- 1 onion, thinly sliced
- 2 cloves garlic, minced

- 1 red bell pepper, thinly sliced

- 1 yellow bell pepper, thinly sliced

- 2 carrots, thinly sliced

- 1 zucchini, thinly sliced

- 1 cup broccoli florets

- 1 cup snap peas

- 3 tablespoons soy sauce

- 1 tablespoon sesame oil

- 1 tablespoon rice vinegar

- 1 tablespoon honey (optional)

- Salt and pepper to taste

- Sesame seeds for garnish (optional)

- Fresh cilantro or parsley for garnish (optional)

Instructions

1. Wash the quinoa under chilly water to eliminate any severe taste. In a pan, consolidate the washed quinoa and water. Heat to the point of boiling, then, at that point, decrease the intensity to low,

cover, and stew for around 15 minutes or until the quinoa is cooked and the water is assimilated. Eliminate the intensity and allow it to sit covered for 5 minutes. Cushion the quinoa with a fork.

2. In a huge skillet or wok, heat the vegetable oil over medium intensity. Add the cut onion and minced garlic and sauté for 2-3 minutes until they become fragrant and somewhat mellowed.

3. Add the cut chime peppers, carrots, zucchini, broccoli florets, and snap peas to the skillet. Pan-sear the vegetables for around 5-7 minutes or until they are delicate and fresh. You can change the cooking time in light of your favoured degree of firmness.

4. In a little bowl, whisk together the soy sauce, sesame oil, rice vinegar, and honey (if utilizing). Pour the sauce over the sautéed vegetables and throw to

equally cover. Season with salt and pepper to taste.

5. Add the cooked quinoa to the skillet and delicately combine everything as one, ensuring the quinoa and vegetables are very much consolidated and covered with the sauce. Cook for an extra 2-3 minutes to warm the quinoa through.

6. Eliminate from intensity and topping with sesame seeds and new cilantro or parsley, whenever wanted.

7. Serve the quinoa and vegetable sautéed food as a principal dish or as a side dish. Appreciate!

Tuna Salad Wrap

Ingredients:

- 1 can of tuna, drained
- 1/4 cup mayonnaise
- 2 tablespoons Dijon mustard

- 1 tablespoon lemon juice

- 1/4 cup diced red onion

- 1/4 cup diced celery

- 1/4 cup diced pickles

- Salt and pepper, to taste

- 4 large flour tortillas

- Lettuce leaves

- Sliced tomatoes

- Sliced cucumbers

- Optional toppings: sliced avocado, shredded cheese

Instructions

1. In a blending bowl, join the depleted fish, mayonnaise, Dijon mustard, and lemon juice. Blend well until all fixings are equitably integrated.

2. Add the diced red onion, celery, and pickles to the fish combination. Mix to join. Season with salt and pepper as indicated by your taste inclinations.

3. Spread out the flour tortillas on a perfect surface. Put lettuce leaves on every tortilla, covering about a portion of the tortilla's surface.

4. Spoon the fish salad combination equitably onto the lettuce leaves on every tortilla.

5. Top the fish salad with cut tomatoes, cucumbers, and some other discretionary garnishes you want, like cut avocado or destroyed cheddar.

6. Overlap the sides of every tortilla towards the middle, then firmly roll the tortilla from the base up, encasing the filling.

7. Slice each wrap down the middle askew, whenever wanted, for simpler taking care of and serving.

8. Serve the fish salad wraps right away, or wrap them firmly in cling wrap or foil for later utilization. They can be

refrigerated for a couple of hours before serving

Lentil Soup with Spinach

Ingredients:

- 1 cup dried lentils
- 1 tablespoon olive oil
- 1 onion, chopped
- 2 cloves garlic, minced
- 2 carrots, diced
- 2 celery stalks, diced
- 1 teaspoon cumin
- 1 teaspoon paprika
- 1/2 teaspoon turmeric
- 4 cups vegetable broth
- 2 cups water
- 1 bay leaf
- 2 cups fresh spinach leaves, chopped
- Salt and pepper to taste
- Lemon wedges for serving

Instructions

1. Wash the lentils under chilly water and put them away.

2. Heat olive oil in a huge pot over medium intensity. Add the hacked onion and minced garlic, and sauté for around 5 minutes until they become clear.

3. Add the diced carrots and celery to the pot and cook for 5 extra minutes, mixing every so often.

4. Mix in the cumin, paprika, and turmeric, and cook for one more moment to permit the flavours to deliver their flavours.

5. Add the washed lentils to the pot, trailed by the vegetable stock, water, and straight leaf. Increment the intensity too high and heat the blend to the point of boiling.

6. When bubbling, lessen the intensity to low, cover the pot, and let the soup stew

for around 25-30 minutes, or until the lentils are delicate.

7. Eliminate the sound leaf from the soup and dispose of it.

8. Mix in the hacked spinach leaves and cook for an extra 2-3 minutes until the spinach shrinks.

9. Season the soup with salt and pepper to taste.

10. Serve the lentil soup hot, embellished with a crush of new lemon juice. Appreciate!

Grilled Vegetable Skewers with Brown Rice

Ingredients:

- 2 cups cooked brown rice
- 2 zucchinis, sliced into rounds

- 2 bell peppers (red, yellow, or green), cut into chunks
- 1 red onion, cut into chunks
- 1 cup cherry tomatoes
- 8-10 button mushrooms
- 2 tablespoons olive oil
- 2 cloves garlic, minced
- 1 teaspoon dried oregano
- 1 teaspoon dried basil
- Salt and pepper to taste
- Wooden skewers, soaked in water for 30 minutes

Instructions

1. Preheat your barbecue to medium-high intensity.
2. In a little bowl, consolidate olive oil, minced garlic, dried oregano, dried basil, salt, and pepper. Blend well to make a marinade.
3.

4. Place the cut zucchinis, chime peppers, red onion lumps, cherry tomatoes, and mushrooms in a huge bowl. Pour the marinade over the vegetables and throw tenderly to equitably cover them. Allow them to marinate for around 15-20 minutes.

5. String the marinated vegetables onto the doused wooden sticks, shifting back and forth between the various vegetables. This will make brilliant and delightful sticks.

6. Put the vegetable sticks on the preheated barbecue and cook for around 8-10 minutes, turning them periodically, until the vegetables are marginally singed and delicate.

7. While the sticks are barbecuing, warm the cooked earthy colored rice in a pan over low intensity or in the microwave.

8. When the vegetable sticks are finished, eliminate them from the barbecue and let them cool for a couple of moments.

9. Serve the barbecued vegetable sticks close by a part of earthy colored rice. You can embellish with new spices like parsley or cilantro whenever wanted.

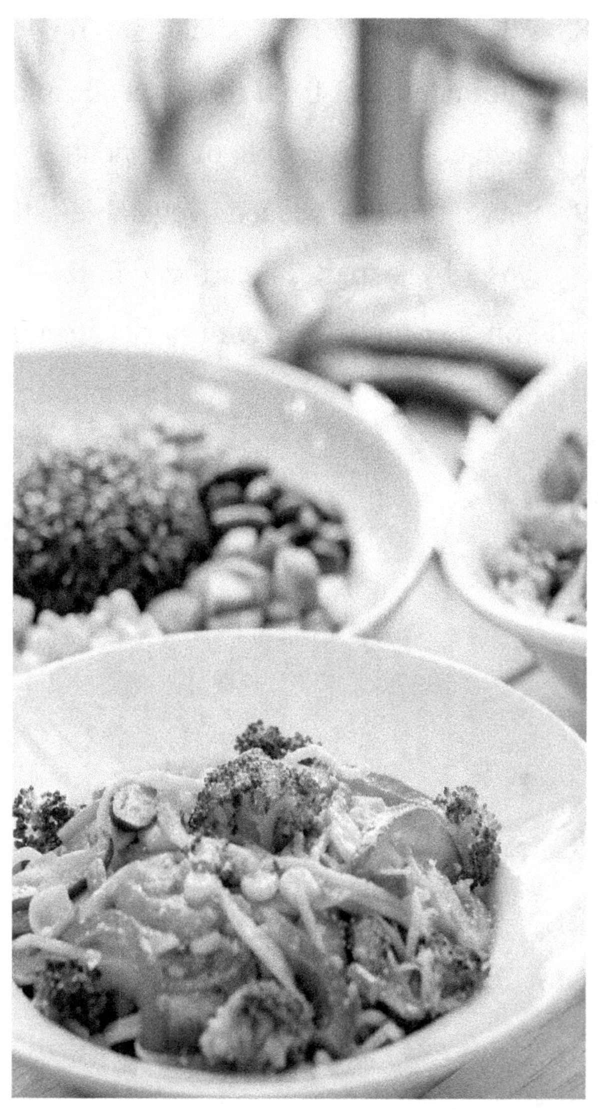

CHAPTER 3: DINNER RECIPES

Baked Salmon with Quinoa and Steamed Vegetables

Ingredients:

- 4 salmon fillets
- 1 cup quinoa
- 2 cups water
- 2 tablespoons olive oil
- 1 lemon, sliced
- 1 teaspoon dried dill
- Salt and pepper to taste
- 2 cups mixed vegetables (such as broccoli, carrots, and snap peas)

Instructions

1. Preheat the stove to 400°F (200°C).

2. Wash the quinoa under cool water to eliminate any harshness. In a medium pan, join the washed quinoa and water. Heat to the point of boiling, then lessen the intensity to low and cover. Allow it to stew for around 15 minutes or until everything the water is ingested. Eliminate from intensity and allow it to sit, covered, for an additional 5 minutes. Cushion the quinoa with a fork.

3. While the quinoa is cooking, set up the salmon. Put the salmon filets on a baking sheet fixed with material paper. Sprinkle olive oil over the filets and season with salt, pepper, and dried dill. Put lemon cuts on top of each filet.

4. Prepare the salmon in the preheated broiler for around 12-15 minutes or until it pieces effectively with a fork and arrives at an inside temperature of 145°F (63°C).

5. Meanwhile, set up the steamed vegetables. Fill a huge pot with around 1 inch of water and spot a liner container inside. Add the blended vegetables to the liner crate. Heat the water to the point of boiling over medium intensity, then, at that point, lessen the intensity to low, cover, and steam the vegetables for around 5-7 minutes, or until they are delicate yet still fresh.

6. When the salmon is cooked and the vegetables are steamed, eliminate them from the intensity.

7. Serve the prepared salmon on a bed of quinoa with steamed vegetables as an afterthought. Press new lemon juice over the salmon filets for added character.

Grilled Chicken Breast with Brown Rice and Roasted Asparagus

Ingredients:

- For the chicken:
- 2 boneless, skinless chicken breasts
- 2 tablespoons olive oil
- 2 cloves of garlic, minced
- 1 teaspoon paprika
- 1 teaspoon dried thyme
- Salt and pepper to taste
- For the brown rice:
- 1 cup brown rice
- 2 cups water or chicken broth
- Salt to taste
- For the roasted asparagus:
- 1 bunch of asparagus, woody ends trimmed
- 2 tablespoons olive oil
- Salt and pepper to taste

Instructions

1. Preheat your barbecue to medium-high intensity.
2. In a little bowl, consolidate olive oil, minced garlic, paprika, dried thyme, salt, and pepper. Blend well.
3. Put the chicken bosoms on a plate and rub the olive oil blend all over them, it are equitably covered to ensure they. Permit the chicken to marinate for around 15-20 minutes.
4. In the interim, flush the earthy-coloured rice under cool water. In a medium-sized pan, consolidate the washed rice, water or chicken stock, and a spot of salt. Heat to the point of boiling, then, at that point, decrease the intensity to low, cover, and stew for around 45 minutes or until the rice is delicate and the fluid is assimilated. Eliminate the intensity and

allow it to sit covered for 5 minutes before lightening with a fork.

5. While the rice is cooking, set up the asparagus. Preheat your stove to 425°F (220°C). Put the managed asparagus on a baking sheet, shower with olive oil, sprinkle with salt and pepper, and throw to cover. Spread the asparagus out in a solitary layer. Cook on the preheated stove for around 10-12 minutes, or until delicate and fresh.

6. Presently, now is the ideal time to barbecue the chicken. Put the marinated chicken bosoms on the preheated barbecue and cook for around 6-8 minutes for each side, or until the inside temperature comes to 165°F (74°C). Cooking times might differ relying on the thickness of the chicken bosoms. Eliminate the chicken from the barbecue

and let it rest for a couple of moments before cutting.

7. Serve the barbecued chicken bosom close by the earthy-coloured rice and broiled asparagus. You can decorate with new spices like parsley or cilantro, whenever wanted.

Turkey Chili with Mixed Salad

Ingredients:

For the Turkey Chili:

- 1 pound ground turkey
- 1 tablespoon olive oil
- 1 medium onion, diced
- 2 cloves garlic, minced
- 1 bell pepper, diced
- 1 jalapeño pepper, seeded and minced (optional, for heat)
- 1 can (14.5 ounces) diced tomatoes

- 1 can (15 ounces) kidney beans, drained and rinsed
- 1 can (15 ounces) black beans, drained and rinsed
- 1 cup chicken broth
- 2 tablespoons chili powder
- 1 tablespoon cumin
- 1 teaspoon paprika
- 1/2 teaspoon oregano
- Salt and pepper to taste
- Optional toppings: shredded cheese, sour cream, chopped cilantro, sliced green onions

For the Mixed Salad:

- 4 cups mixed salad greens
- 1 cup cherry tomatoes, halved
- 1 cucumber, diced
- 1/2 red onion, thinly sliced
- 1/4 cup feta cheese, crumbled
- 2 tablespoons balsamic vinegar
- 2 tablespoons olive oil

- Salt and pepper to taste

Instructions

1. In an enormous pot or Dutch broiler, heat the olive oil over medium intensity. Add the ground turkey and cook until caramelized, separating it with a spoon or spatula.

2. Add the diced onion, minced garlic, ringer pepper, and jalapeño pepper (if utilizing) to the pot. Cook for around 5 minutes until the vegetables relax.

3. Mix in the diced tomatoes, kidney beans, dark beans, chicken stock, stew powder, cumin, paprika, oregano, salt, and pepper. Carry the combination to a stew.

4. Lessen the intensity to low, cover the pot, and let the bean stew for 30-40 minutes to permit the flavours to merge. Mix sometimes.

5. While the bean stew is stewing, set up the blended serving of mixed greens. In a huge serving of mixed greens bowl, consolidate the blended serving of mixed greens, cherry tomatoes, cucumber, red onion, and disintegrated feta cheddar.

6. In a little bowl, whisk together the balsamic vinegar, olive oil, salt, and pepper to make the serving of mixed greens dressing.

7. Pour the dressing over the plate of mixed greens fixings and throw tenderly to cover.

8. When the stew is prepared, taste and change the flavouring if necessary. Serve the turkey stew hot in bowls, and top with discretionary garnishes like destroyed cheddar, harsh cream, cleaved cilantro, or cut green onions.

9. Serve the turkey bean stew close by the blended plate of mixed greens for an invigorating differentiation. Appreciate!

Stir-Fried Shrimp with Brown Rice Noodles and Stir-Fried Vegetables

Ingredients:

- 8 ounces brown rice noodles
- 1 pound shrimp, peeled and deveined
- 2 tablespoons soy sauce
- 1 tablespoon oyster sauce
- 1 tablespoon sesame oil
- 2 cloves garlic, minced
- 1 teaspoon grated ginger
- 1 red bell pepper, thinly sliced
- 1 medium carrot, thinly sliced
- 1 cup snap peas, ends trimmed
- 1 cup broccoli florets
- 2 green onions, chopped
- 2 tablespoons vegetable oil

- Salt and pepper to taste

Instructions

1. Cook the earthy-coloured rice noodles as indicated by the bundle guidelines. Channel and put away.

2. In a little bowl, whisk together the soy sauce, clam sauce, and sesame oil. Put away.

3. Heat 1 tablespoon of vegetable oil in a huge skillet or wok over medium-high intensity. Add the shrimp and cook for 2-3 minutes until pink and cooked through. Eliminate the shrimp from the skillet and put it away.

4. In a similar skillet, add the excess tablespoon of vegetable oil. Add the garlic and ginger, and sautéed food for around 1 moment until fragrant.

5. Add the ringer pepper, carrot, snap peas, and broccoli to the skillet. Pan-sear for

3-4 minutes until the vegetables are delicate and fresh.

6. Return the cooked shrimp to the skillet and pour the sauce over the shrimp and vegetables. Pan-sear for an extra 1-2 minutes until everything is all around covered in the sauce.

7. Add the cooked earthy-coloured rice noodles to the skillet and throw to join with the shrimp and vegetables. Cook for another 1-2 minutes until the noodles are warmed through.

8. Season with salt and pepper to taste. Mix in the hacked green onions.

9. Eliminate the intensity and serve the sautéed shrimp, earthy-coloured rice noodles, and vegetables hot. Appreciate!

Baked Chicken Thighs with Sweet Potato

Ingredients:

- 4 bone-in, skin-on chicken thighs
- 2 medium sweet potatoes, peeled and cut into cubes
- 2 tablespoons olive oil
- 2 cloves garlic, minced
- 1 teaspoon paprika
- 1/2 teaspoon dried thyme
- 1/2 teaspoon dried rosemary
- Salt and black pepper to taste
- Fresh parsley for garnish

Instructions

1. Preheat your broiler to 400°F (200°C).
2. In a little bowl, combine as one the minced garlic, paprika, dried thyme, dried rosemary, salt, and dark pepper.

3. Put the chicken thighs on a baking sheet fixed with material paper. Shower 1 tablespoon of olive oil over the chicken thighs, then sprinkle the flavour combination equally on the two sides of the chicken. Rub the flavours into the chicken to guarantee they are all around covered.

4. In a different bowl, throw the yam shapes with the leftover 1 tablespoon of olive oil and a touch of salt and pepper.

5. Orchestrate the yam 3D shapes around the chicken thighs on the baking sheet.

6. Place the baking sheet in the preheated broiler and prepare for 35-40 minutes, or until the chicken is cooked through and the yams are delicate. The chicken ought to have an inner temperature of 165°F (74°C).

7. Once cooked, eliminate the baking sheet from the stove and let the chicken rest for a couple of moments.

8. Serve the prepared chicken thighs with the cooked yams. Embellish with new parsley for added newness and flavour.

Mash and Steamed Green Beans

Ingredients:

- 4 large potatoes
- 1/2 cup milk
- 4 tablespoons butter
- Salt, to taste
- Pepper, to taste
- 1 pound fresh green beans
- Water for steaming

Instructions

1. Strip the potatoes and cut them into little pieces. Wash them under chilly water to eliminate any overabundance of starch.

2. In a huge pot, heat water to the point of boiling. Add the potato pieces and cook them until they are fork-delicate, around 15-20 minutes.

3. While the potatoes are cooking, set up the green beans. Trim the closures and wash them under cool water.

4. Fill a liner pot or a huge pan with two or three creeps of water. Place a liner bushel inside, ensuring the water doesn't contact the lower part of the bin.

5. Heat the water to the point of boiling over medium intensity. Add the green beans to the liner crate, cover, and steam them for around 5-7 minutes or until they are delicate yet at the same time hold a slight freshness.

6. When the potatoes are cooked, channel them well and return them to the pot.

7. Add milk, margarine, salt, and pepper to the pot with the potatoes. Squash the potatoes utilizing a potato masher or a fork until they arrive at your ideal consistency. If you favour a creamier surface, you can utilize a hand blender or a blender.

8. Taste the pureed potatoes and change the flavouring if necessary.

9. Move the pureed potatoes to a serving dish.

10. Channel the steamed green beans and wipe them off delicately with a paper towel.

11. Organize the green beans close by the pureed potatoes on the serving dish.

12. Serve the pound and steamed green beans as a side dish to go with your fundamental course.

Vegetable Curry with Cauliflower Rice

Ingredients:

For the Vegetable Curry:

- 1 tablespoon vegetable oil
- 1 onion, diced
- 2 cloves garlic, minced
- 1 tablespoon curry powder
- 1 teaspoon ground cumin
- 1 teaspoon ground coriander
- 1/2 teaspoon turmeric
- 1/4 teaspoon cayenne pepper (optional, for heat)
- 1 bell pepper, diced
- 2 carrots, sliced
- 1 zucchini, diced
- 1 cup cauliflower florets
- 1 cup broccoli florets
- 1 can (14 ounces) coconut milk
- 1 cup vegetable broth
- Salt and pepper to taste

- Fresh cilantro, chopped (for garnish)
- For the Cauliflower Rice:
- 1 head of cauliflower
- 1 tablespoon vegetable oil
- Salt and pepper to taste

Instructions

1. Set up the Cauliflower Rice:
2. Cut the cauliflower into florets and wash them completely.
3. Place the florets in a food processor and heartbeat until they look like rice grains.
4. Heat the vegetable oil in an enormous skillet over medium intensity.
5. Add the cauliflower rice to the skillet and sauté for 5-7 minutes, until delicate.
6. Season with salt and pepper to taste. Put away.
7. Set up the Vegetable Curry:
8. Heat the vegetable oil in an enormous pot or skillet over medium intensity.

9. Add the diced onion and minced garlic to the pot and sauté until the onion becomes clear.

10. Add the curry powder, cumin, coriander, turmeric, and cayenne pepper (if utilizing) to the pot. Mix well to cover the onions and garlic with the flavours.

11. Add the diced ringer pepper, cut carrots, diced zucchini, cauliflower florets, and broccoli florets to the pot. Mix to join with the flavours.

12. Pour in the coconut milk and vegetable stock. Carry the combination to a stew.

13. Decrease the intensity to low, cover the pot, and let the curry stew for 15-20 minutes, or until the vegetables are delicate.

14. Season with salt and pepper to taste.

15. Serve:

16. Spoon the cauliflower rice onto plates or bowls.

17. Scoop the vegetable curry over the cauliflower rice.

18. Decorate with new slashed cilantro.

19. Partake in your heavenly Vegetable Curry with Cauliflower Rice!

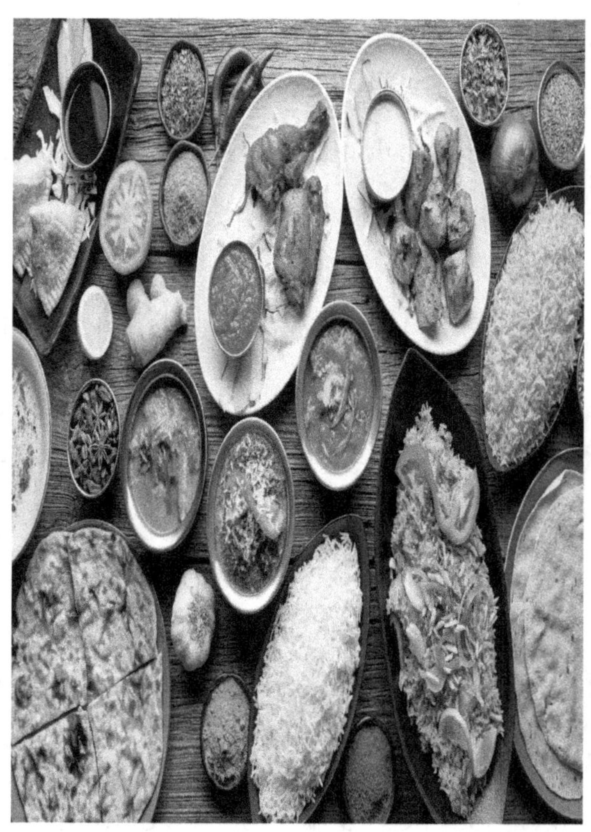

CHAPTER 4: SNACKS AND APPETIZERS

Greek yogurt with fresh berries

Ingredients:

- 1 cup Greek yogurt
- 1 cup mixed fresh berries (such as strawberries, blueberries, raspberries)
- 1 tablespoon honey (optional)
- 1/4 cup granola or muesli (optional)
- Fresh mint leaves for garnish (optional)

Instructions

1. Wash the new berries completely and wipe them off with a paper towel.
2. If the berries are enormous, you can cut them into more modest pieces. Leave more modest berries, similar to blueberries, in entirety.

3. In a bowl, add the Greek yoghurt and honey (if utilizing). Blend well until the honey is equitably integrated into the yoghurt.

4. Add the new berries to the bowl with the yoghurt. Delicately overlap them in, taking consideration not to smash the berries.

5. Whenever wanted, sprinkle granola or muesli on top of the yoghurt and berries for added crunch and surface.

6. Decorate with new mint leaves for a pop of variety and newness.

7. Serve right away and appreciate!

Cucumber and cream cheese roll-ups

Ingredients:

- 4 large cucumbers

- 8 ounces (226 grams) cream cheese, softened

- 1 tablespoon fresh dill, finely chopped
- 1 tablespoon fresh chives, finely chopped
- Salt and black pepper to taste

Instructions

1. Begin by setting up the cucumbers. Wash them completely and trim off the finishes. Utilizing a vegetable peeler or a mandoline slicer, cut the cucumbers longwise into slim, long strips.

2. In a blending bowl, consolidate the relaxed cream cheddar, new dill, new chives, salt, and dark pepper. Mix well until every one of the fixings is uniformly consolidated.

3. Lay the cucumber cuts level on a perfect surface or cutting board. Spread a fair layer of the cream cheddar blend onto every cucumber cut, covering the whole surface.

4. When the cream cheddar is spread, cautiously roll up every cucumber cut, beginning from one end and rolling firmly. Secure the roll-ups with toothpicks if necessary to keep them set up.

5. Rehash the cycle until all the cucumber cuts are utilized and you have a plate of wonderful roll-ups.

6. Serve the cucumber and cream cheddar roll-ups right away or refrigerate them for around 30 minutes to permit the flavours to merge and the rolls to set.

7. Alternatively, you can embellish the roll-ups with extra new dill or chives before serving.

Celery sticks with almond butter

Ingredients:

- 4-6 stalks of celery

- 1/2 cup almond butter

- Optional toppings: sliced almonds, raisins, or chia seeds (for garnish)

Instructions:

1. To get rid of any dirt or debris, thoroughly wash the celery stalks in cold water. With a fresh towel, pat them dry.

2. Remove the celery stalks' rough ends and green tips. Create celery sticks by cutting the stalks into 3–4 inch-long segments.

3. To soften the almond butter, place it in a bowl that may be heated in the microwave for 20 to 30 seconds. As an alternative, you might let the almond butter sit at room temperature for some time to make it easier to spread.

4. Take a celery stick, and generously smear almond butter around the stalk's inner curve. Spread the almond butter

evenly using the back of a spoon or a butter knife.

5. Spread almond butter on each of the remaining celery sticks and repeat the procedure.

6. Sliced almonds, raisins, or chia seeds may be added as a finishing touch to give the almond butter a lovely garnish and more texture.

7. Place the prepared celery sticks on a dish or serving tray.

8. As a tasty appetizer or nutritious snack, serve it right away.

Turkey lettuce wraps with avocado

Ingredients:

- 1 lb ground turkey
- 2 tablespoons olive oil
- 1 small onion, diced
- 2 cloves garlic, minced

- 1 teaspoon ground cumin

- 1 teaspoon chili powder

- 1/2 teaspoon paprika

- Salt and pepper to taste

- 1 avocado, sliced

- Juice of 1 lime

- 8 large lettuce leaves (such as Bibb or iceberg)

- Optional toppings: chopped tomatoes, shredded cheese, cilantro, salsa, sour cream

Instructions:

1. A big skillet with medium heat is used to heat the olive oil. Add the minced garlic and onion, and cook until the onion is transparent and aromatic.

2. When the ground turkey is brown and cooked through, add it to the skillet and heat it, breaking it up with a wooden spoon.

3. To the skillet, add the ground cumin, chilli powder, paprika, salt, and pepper. Stir well to coat the turkey with the seasonings.

4. The turkey mixture should simmer for a further five minutes on low heat to enable the flavours to mingle. If necessary, taste and adjust the spices.

5. Slices of avocado and lime juice should be mashed together in a small dish to get a creamy texture.

6. The lettuce leaves should be washed, dried, and then spread out on a level surface.

7. Place a spoonful of mashed avocado on top of each lettuce leaf after spooning the turkey mixture into the leaf's middle.

8. Add any additional toppings, such as sour cream, diced tomatoes, shredded cheese, cilantro, salsa, or salsa if you want.

9. To make a wrap, roll up the lettuce leaves and tuck the sides in as you go.

10. Serve the turkey lettuce wraps right away with avocado and take a bite.

Oven-baked sweet potato fries (in moderation)

Ingredients:

- 2 medium-sized sweet potatoes
- 2 tablespoons olive oil
- 1 teaspoon paprika
- 1/2 teaspoon garlic powder
- 1/2 teaspoon salt
- 1/4 teaspoon black pepper

Instructions:

1. A baking sheet should be lightly greased or lined with parchment paper and heated to 425°F (220°C).

2. The sweet potatoes should be carefully cleaned before being dried with a kitchen

towel. For extra texture and nutrition, keep the skin on.

3. Sweet potatoes should be sliced into thin, even slices. For a crispy texture, try to maintain a thickness of around 1/4 inch. You may trim them to any desired length.

4. Olive oil, paprika, garlic powder, salt, and black pepper should all be combined in a big bowl. Mix well until the spices are distributed equally.

5. Swish the sweet potato strips about in the bowl to evenly distribute the spice mixture. Make sure each strip has a uniform coating.

6. On the baking sheet that has been prepared, arrange the coated sweet potato strips in a single layer. The fries should not be packed too tightly as this might prevent them from being crispy.

7. The baking sheet should be placed in the preheated oven and baked for 20 to 25

minutes, or until the sweet potato fries are crispy and golden brown. To ensure consistent cooking, flip them halfway during the baking period.

8. When the sweet potato fries are done, take them out of the oven and let them cool for a while.

9. The oven-baked sweet potato fries make a delightful side dish or snack when you serve them right away. They may be eaten alone or with your preferred dipping sauce, such as ketchup, garlic aioli, or hot mayo.

Sliced apples with natural peanut butter

Ingredients:

- 2 medium-sized apples (any variety you prefer)

- Natural peanut butter (smooth or crunchy)
- Optional toppings: honey, cinnamon, raisins, granola, or chopped nuts

Instructions:

1. Under running water, thoroughly wash the apples. With a fresh kitchen towel, pat them dry.
2. Using an apple corer or a sharp knife, core the apples. Eliminate the seeds and stalks.
3. Using a sharp knife, cut the apples into round, thin slices. If you'd like, you may also cut them into wedges.
4. Place the apple slices on separate plates or a serving dish.
5. Each apple slice should have a teaspoon of natural peanut butter applied to it. The quantity of peanut butter may be changed to suit your tastes.

6. For an optional touch of sweetness, drizzle a little honey over the peanut butter.

7. If desired, add a little cinnamon to the peanut butter. The apples will acquire a warm and fragrant taste as a result.

8. You may top the peanut butter with other ingredients like raisins, oats, or chopped nuts for more texture and taste.

9. Sliced apples and natural peanut butter make a tasty and nutritious snack. Serve right now and enjoy!

Spinach and feta stuffed mushrooms

Ingredients:

- 12 large mushrooms
- 2 cups fresh spinach, chopped
- 1/2 cup crumbled feta cheese
- 2 cloves garlic, minced

- 2 tablespoons olive oil
- 1/4 teaspoon salt
- 1/4 teaspoon black pepper
- 1/4 teaspoon dried oregano
- 1/4 teaspoon dried thyme
- 1/4 cup grated Parmesan cheese (optional, for topping)

Instructions:

1. Set the oven's temperature to 375°F (190°C). Use cooking spray or a little olive oil to grease a baking pan.

2. The mushroom stems should be cut off and kept aside. Place the mushroom caps with the gills facing up in the prepared baking dish.

3. Chop the mushroom stems finely. Olive oil should be heated in a large pan over medium heat. Add the minced garlic, dry thyme, dried oregano, and sliced mushroom stems. Sauté the mushrooms

for 3 to 4 minutes, or until they are soft and any liquid has disappeared.

4. When the spinach has begun to wilt, add the chopped spinach to the pan and simmer for an additional 2 to 3 minutes. To taste, add salt and black pepper to the food.

5. After turning off the heat, add the feta cheese crumbles and stir until fully blended.

6. Fill every mushroom cap to the brim with the spinach and feta mixture.

7. If more cheese is required, top the filled mushrooms with grated Parmesan cheese.

8. Bake for 15 to 20 minutes in a preheated oven, or until the cheese is melted and the top is gently browned.

9. After cooking, take the mushrooms out of the oven and allow them cool before serving.

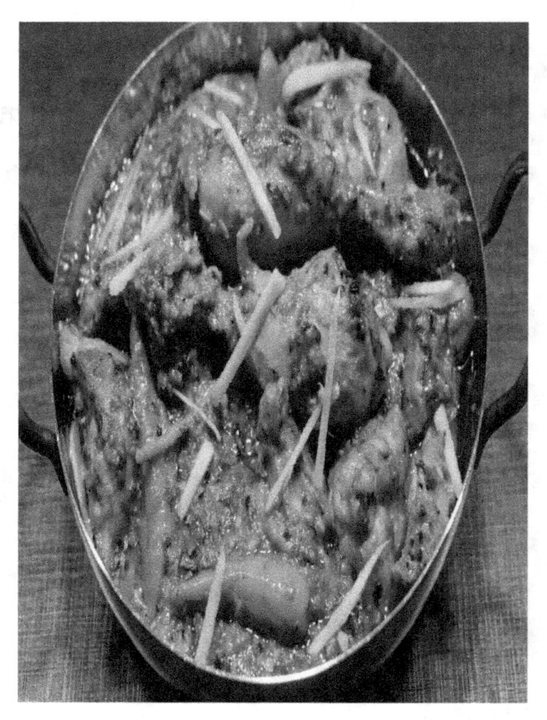

CHAPTER 5: DESSERT RECIPES

Sugar-free Jello

Ingredients:

- 1 package (0.3 ounces or 8 grams) sugar-free flavored gelatin (any flavor of your choice)
- 1 cup boiling water
- 1 cup cold water

Instructions:

1. Fill a medium bowl with the sugar-free flavoured gelatin from the packet.
2. In the basin containing the gelatin, pour the boiling water. Until the gelatin powder is entirely dissolved, stir continually.

3. Stir the dish well after adding the cold water.

4. For approximately 5 minutes, let the mixture stand at room temperature to gently cool.

5. You might choose to skim any froth that has developed on top of the gelatin mixture.

6. Fill individual serving dishes or a larger serving dish with the gelatin mixture.

7. Refrigerate the bowls or dishes for at least 4 hours, or until the gelatin has set.

8. When the gelatin has hardened, you can either serve it plain or top it with fresh fruit or sugar-free whipped cream for taste and texture enhancement.

9. Enjoy your tasty homemade Jello that is devoid of sugar!

Berry Parfait

Ingredients:

- 1 cup fresh mixed berries (such as strawberries, blueberries, raspberries)
- 2 tablespoons granulated sugar
- 1 teaspoon lemon juice
- 1 cup Greek yogurt
- 1/2 cup granola
- Honey (optional)
- Fresh mint leaves for garnish (optional)

Instructions:

1. The fresh mixed berries, granulated sugar, and lemon juice should all be combined in a medium bowl. Gently toss the berries in the sugar-lemon juice mixture to coat them. To enable the flavours to merge and the berries to release their juices, let them rest for about 10 minutes.

2. Layer the berry mixture, Greek yoghurt, and granola in serving glasses or bowls. The bottom layer should be the berry combination, then come to a layer of Greek yoghurt, and finally a coating of granola. Continue layering the ingredients until you've used them all up, finishing with a final layer of Greek yoghurt and a dusting of oats on top.

3. If you want it to be sweeter, drizzle honey on top. This phase is optional and may be customized to suit your tastes.

4. If desired, garnish with fresh mint leaves to add colour and freshness.

5. Enjoy this hydrating and wholesome Berry Parfait right now!

Coconut Macaroons

Ingredients:

- 2 2/3 cups shredded coconut (unsweetened)
- 1/2 cup granulated sugar
- 3 tablespoons all-purpose flour
- 1/4 teaspoon salt
- 4 large egg whites
- 1 teaspoon vanilla extract

Instructions:

1. Set your oven's temperature to 325 °F (160 °C). Use silicone baking mats or parchment paper to line a baking pan.
2. Combine the flour, salt, sugar, and coconut flakes in a large mixing basin. Mix well until all components are spread equally.
3. The egg whites should be whipped until foamy in a separate basin. You may whisk by hand or with a low-speed electric mixer.

4. Add the vanilla essence and foaming egg whites to the coconut mixture. Gently fold everything together until the egg whites are applied evenly to the coconut. Watch carefully not to combine too much.

5. Drop rounded mounds of the coconut mixture onto the prepared baking sheet using a tablespoon or a tiny cookie scoop. They should be roughly 1 inch apart.

6. The macaroons should be baked in the preheated oven for about 20 minutes, or until the edges start to become golden. Touching the tops should feel somewhat stiff.

7. The macaroons should cool on the baking sheet for a few minutes after the baking sheet is taken out of the oven. After that, move them to a wire rack to finish cooling.

8. Optional: If you'd like to add flavour and decoration to the cooled macaroons, melt some chocolate (milk, dark, or white) and pour it on top. Before serving, give the chocolate time to set.

9. Your coconut macaroons are prepared for consumption after they have cooled and any optional chocolate has hardened. For up to a week, keep them at room temperature in an airtight container.

Grilled Pineapple

Ingredients:

- 1 ripe pineapple
- 2 tablespoons honey
- 1 tablespoon lime juice
- 1 teaspoon ground cinnamon
- Vanilla ice cream (optional, for serving)
- Fresh mint leaves (optional, for garnish

Instructions:

1. Heat your grill to a moderately hot setting.

2. Remove the pineapple's outer shell and core to prepare it. Depending on your preference, cut the pineapple into slices or spears.

3. Combine the honey, lime juice, and ground cinnamon in a small bowl. To make a glaze for the pineapple, thoroughly combine.

4. Apply the glaze equally on both sides of the pineapple spears or slices by brushing.

5. Grill the pineapple over direct fire for 3 to 4 minutes on each side, or until grill marks appear and the pineapple is well cooked. Avoid overcooking the pineapple, as it might get mushy.

6. Grilled pineapple should be taken from the grill and placed on a serving plate.

7. For a pleasant taste contrast, serve the grilled pineapple by itself or with a dollop of vanilla ice cream. Fresh mint leaves may be used as a garnish to give more freshness.

8. While it's still warm, savour your wonderful grilled pineapple right away!

Almond Flour Brownies

Ingredients:

- 1 cup almond flour
- 1/2 cup cocoa powder
- 1/2 teaspoon baking soda
- 1/4 teaspoon salt
- 1/2 cup unsalted butter, melted
- 1/2 cup honey or maple syrup
- 2 large eggs
- 1 teaspoon vanilla extract
- 1/2 cup dark chocolate chips

Instructions:

1. Turn on the oven to 350 °F (175 °C). A square baking pan should be greased or lined with parchment paper.

2. Mix the almond flour, cocoa powder, baking soda, and salt in a medium basin. Place aside.

3. Butter that has been melted and honey (or maple syrup) should be well blended in a different, big bowl. One at a time, whisk thoroughly after each addition of the eggs. Add the vanilla essence and stir.

4. Stirring occasionally, add the dry ingredients in small amounts to the wet components. Watch carefully not to combine too much.

5. A few of the dark chocolate chips may be saved for topping if preferred. Fold them in.

6. Use a spatula to distribute the batter uniformly after pouring it onto the

baking dish that has been prepared. Top with the chocolate chips you set aside.

7. Bake for 25 to 30 minutes in the preheated oven, or until a toothpick inserted in the middle emerges with a few moist crumbs attached.

8. After taking the brownies out of the oven, let them cool for approximately 10 minutes in the baking dish. After that, move them to a wire rack and allow them to cool completely before cutting them into squares.

9. Serve the brownies made with almond flour alone or with a dollop of ice cream, powdered sugar, or another preferred garnish. Enjoy!

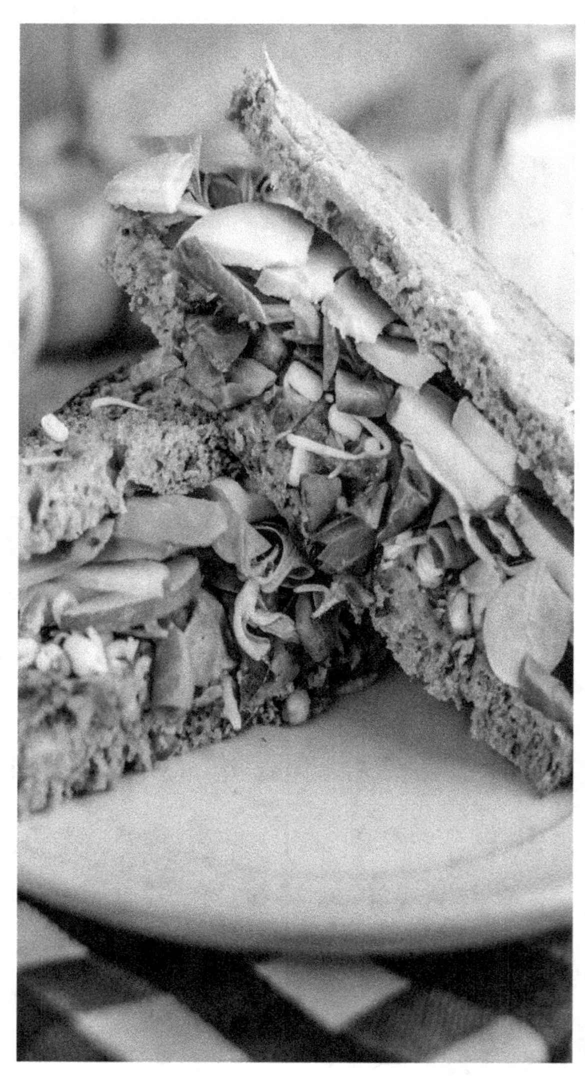

CHAPTER 6 BEVERAGES

Herbal tea

Ingredients:

- 2 cups water
- 1 tablespoon dried chamomile flowers
- 1 tablespoon dried peppermint leaves
- 1 tablespoon dried lemon balm leaves
- 1 teaspoon dried lavender flowers (optional)
- Honey or lemon (optional, for taste)

Instructions:

1. In a pot or kettle, bring the water to a boil.

2. Make your herbal tea mix while the water is heating. Combine the dried chamomile flowers, dried peppermint leaves, dried lemon balm leaves, and dried lavender flowers (if using) in a tea infuser or a small dish. To achieve

uniform dispersion, thoroughly mix them.

3. Remove the water from the heat after it comes to a rolling boil and let it cool for a minute.

4. In a teapot or other heat-resistant container, pour the herbal tea mixture. To fully cover the herbs, pour the boiling water over them.

5. Allow the herbs to soak in the boiling water for 5 to 7 minutes while covering the teapot or container. For a stronger or milder taste, you may change the steeping period to your liking.

6. After steeping, filter the herbal tea into individual teacups using a fine-mesh sieve or a tea strainer.

7. For a hint of sweetness or zesty taste, add honey or lemon after tasting the herbal tea. To blend, thoroughly stir.

8. Enjoy the herbal tea's calming and fragrant properties while it is still warm by serving it.

Unsweetened almond milk

Ingredients:

- 1 cup raw almonds
- 4 cups filtered water
- Optional: pinch of salt

Instructions:

1. Almonds should be placed in a basin and covered with water to soak. Allow them to soak for at least eight hours or overnight. Almonds are softened during this procedure, which facilitates blending.

2. After soaking the almonds, drain them and give them a thorough rinsing with

fresh water. This procedure aids in purging any contaminants.

3. Almonds and water to be blended: Add 4 cups of filtered water to the soaked almonds in a blender. Add a dash of salt to taste, if you like. For two to three minutes on high speed, blend the ingredients until it is smooth and creamy.

4. Set a fine-mesh strainer or nut milk bag over a large basin or pitcher to strain the mixture. Pour the almond mixture into the bag or sieve gradually so that the pulp is trapped and the liquid may flow through.

5. Squeeze out any residual milk by gathering the corners of the bag or strainer after the bulk of the liquid has been filtered through. Avoid using too much pressure as this might result in the milk becoming gritty.

6. Pour the newly strained almond milk into a clean glass jar or container to transfer and store. It may be kept in the fridge for up to four or five days. Shake well before each usage since separation is expected.

7. Customize your almond milk as you like. If you'd like, you may flavour it with things like vanilla essence or sweeten it with things like honey or dates, which are natural sweeteners. To find the flavour that best suits your palate, explore.

Vegetable juice

Ingredients:

- 2 large carrots
- 1 cucumber
- 2 stalks of celery
- 1 small beetroot

- 1 handful of spinach
- 1 small piece of ginger (optional)
- 1 lemon

Instructions:

1. To get rid of any dirt or contaminants, thoroughly rinse all the veggies under cold water.
2. If preferred, peel the carrots and beets to get rid of the outer skin.
3. To easily put the veggies into your juicer, cut them into little pieces or slices.
4. Peel and chop whatever ginger you use into tiny pieces.
5. Eliminate the seeds by halving the lemon.
6. Put your juicer in the middle of all the chopped veggies, ginger, and lemon.
7. Start the juicer, then run it through all the components to get smooth juice.

8. To get rid of any pulp or fibrous parts, you may filter the juice using a fine-mesh strainer.

9. In a glass or other container, pour the vegetable juice and give it a good swirl.

10. The juice may be chilled for later use or served right away over ice.

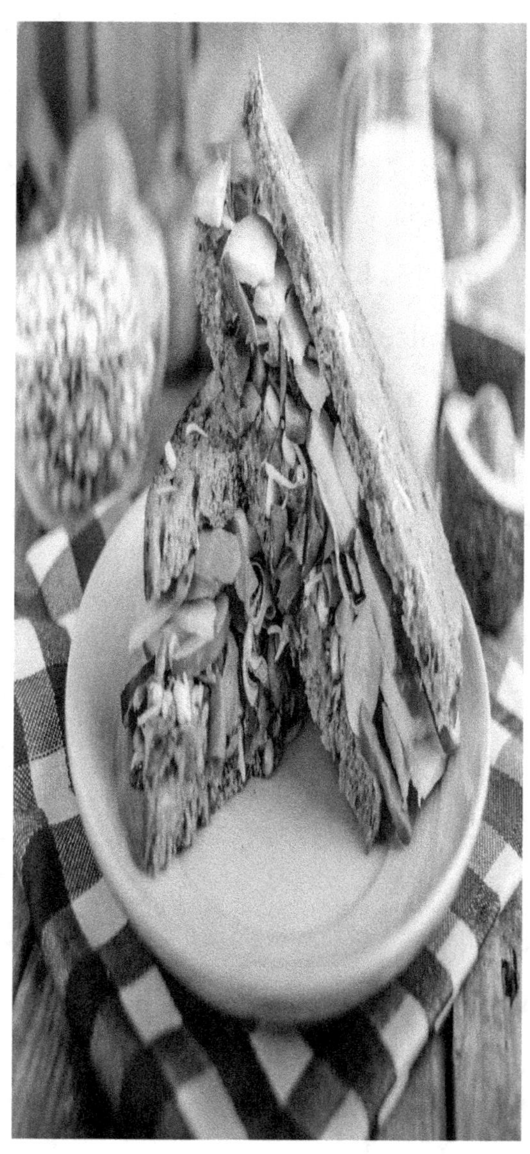

CHAPTER 7: SMOOTHIES

Berry Blast Smoothie

Ingredients:

- 1 cup mixed berries (strawberries, blueberries, raspberries)
- 1 ripe banana
- 1 cup Greek yogurt
- 1/2 cup orange juice
- 1/4 cup almond milk (or any other milk of your choice)
- 1 tablespoon honey or agave syrup (optional, for added sweetness)
- Ice cubes (optional, for a colder smoothie)

Instructions:

1. Wash the berries thoroughly and remove any stems or leaves. If using larger berries like strawberries, you can slice

them into smaller pieces for easier blending.

2. Peel the ripe banana and break it into chunks.

3. In a blender, add the mixed berries, banana chunks, Greek yoghurt, orange juice, almond milk, and honey (if using).

4. If you prefer a colder smoothie, you can also add a handful of ice cubes to the blender.

5. Blend all the ingredients on high speed until you achieve a smooth and creamy texture. If needed, you can add a little more almond milk or orange juice to adjust the consistency.

6. Once blended, taste the smoothie and adjust the sweetness by adding more honey if desired.

7. Pour the Berry Blast Smoothie into glasses and serve immediately. You can

garnish it with a few fresh berries or a sprig of mint if you like.

8. Enjoy your delicious and refreshing Berry Blast Smoothie!

Green Power Smoothie

Ingredients:

- 2 cups spinach leaves
- 1 ripe banana
- 1 green apple, cored and chopped
- 1/2 cucumber, peeled and chopped
- 1/2 lemon, juiced
- 1/2 cup fresh parsley leaves
- 1/2 cup almond milk (or any other plant-based milk)
- 1 tablespoon chia seeds
- Ice cubes (optional)

Instructions:

1. The spinach leaves should be carefully washed before being put in a blender.

2. The green apple, cucumber, and parsley leaves should all be diced before being added to the blender with the peeled banana.

3. Juice from the lemon half should be squeezed and added to the blender.

4. Chia seeds and almond milk should also be added to the blender.

5. If you'd like, you may add some ice cubes to the smoothie to make it cooler and more energizing.

6. Until the mixture is smooth and creamy, combine all the ingredients and blend at high speed. If necessary, you may increase the thickness by adding a bit more almond milk.

7. After it has been combined, taste the smoothie and, if necessary, add

additional lemon juice or a spoonful of honey to sweeten it.

8. The Green Power Smoothie should be poured into glasses and served right away.

Tropical Delight Smoothie

Ingredients:

- 1 ripe banana
- 1 cup frozen mango chunks
- 1/2 cup pineapple chunks (fresh or frozen)
- 1/2 cup coconut milk
- 1/2 cup orange juice
- 1 tablespoon honey (optional, for added sweetness)
- 1/2 cup ice cubes (optional, for a colder smoothie)
- Fresh mint leaves for garnish (optional)

Instructions:

1. Bananas should be peeled and cut into pieces. Blend the banana pieces in a food processor.

2. The frozen pineapple and mango pieces should be added to the blender.

3. Add the orange juice and coconut milk.

4. If more sweetness is wanted, you may add a spoonful of honey to the blender.

5. Add some ice cubes to the blender if you'd like your smoothie to be cooler.

6. On high speed, combine all the ingredients until they are smooth and creamy. You may add a bit extra coconut milk or orange juice to smooth down the mixture if it is too thick.

7. Stop mixing the smoothie when it reaches the correct consistency, and then pour it into a tall glass.

8. If preferred, add a sprig of fresh mint leaves as a garnish to the smoothie to bring in some colour and freshness.

9. Before consuming the smoothie, give it a moderate stir.

10. Take a sip and enjoy the smoothie's tropical tastes. Bananas, mango, pineapple, and coconut, with a tinge of citrus from the orange juice, make up this delectable concoction.

11. Immediately serve the Tropical Delight Smoothie and enjoy it as a light snack, breakfast, or dessert.

Cinnamon Apple Pie Smoothie

Ingredients:

- 1 large apple, cored and chopped
- 1 ripe banana
- 1 cup unsweetened almond milk (or milk of your choice)

- 1/2 cup plain Greek yogurt

- 2 tablespoons rolled oats

- 1 tablespoon honey or maple syrup

- 1/2 teaspoon ground cinnamon

- 1/4 teaspoon vanilla extract

- 1 cup ice cubes

Instructions:

1. Blend the apple, banana, rolled oats, honey or maple syrup, cinnamon powder, and vanilla extract in a blender. Add the almond milk and Greek yoghurt last.

2. Blend everything at a high speed until it's smooth and well-combined.

3. When the smoothie is thick and creamy, add the ice cubes and keep churning.

4. After tasting the smoothie, adjust the sweetness or cinnamon to your liking.

5. Pour the smoothie into glasses and, if preferred, garnish with a little additional cinnamon.

6. Enjoy your reviving Cinnamon Apple Pie Smoothie right now!

Creamy Banana Nut Smoothie

Ingredients:

- 2 ripe bananas
- 1 cup almond milk (or any milk of your choice)
- 1/4 cup Greek yogurt
- 2 tablespoons almond butter
- 1 tablespoon honey (optional, for added sweetness)
- 1/4 teaspoon vanilla extract
- 1/4 cup chopped nuts (such as walnuts or almonds)
- Ice cubes (optional, for a chilled smoothie)

Instructions:

1. Bananas should be peeled and cut into smaller pieces.

2. Blend the banana chunks in a food processor.

3. Blender ingredients should include almond milk, Greek yoghurt, almond butter, honey (if used), and vanilla extract.

4. Blend each item until it is creamy and smooth.

5. For a cooled smoothie, if preferred, add some ice cubes to the blender and process once more.

6. Pour the smoothie into cups for serving.

7. The smoothie should have chopped nuts on it.

8. If desired, you may also add a piece of banana or a drizzle of honey as a garnish.

9. Enjoy the smooth, creamy banana-nut smoothie right now!

Conclusion

Additional Resources

Jessica G farmer, author of "The Renal Diet Cookbook for Diabetics: Manage Diabetes and Kidney Disease with Delicious, Kidney-Friendly Recipes": Particularly designed for those with diabetes and renal illness, this cookbook. It offers a variety of delectable meals that are low in sodium, phosphorus, and potassium and suited for those on a renal diet. The book also offers useful advice on how to control renal disease and diabetes via dietary changes.

- Lasselle Press's "The Complete Kidney Health Cookbook for Diabetics: Simple and Delicious Recipes for Healthy Kidneys": This cookbook provides a selection of quick-to-make dishes that support kidney function and are suitable for diabetics. It comprises foods that are tasty and filling while being low in salt, phosphorus, and potassium. The book also offers crucial pointers and advice for controlling renal disease and diabetes.

- American Diabetes Association (ADA): People with diabetes may find a wealth of information on the ADA website at www.diabetes.org. Although it may not be directly geared toward renal diets, it provides a lot of knowledge about managing diabetes, eating well, and meal planning. The website offers recipes, menu suggestions, and advice on carbohydrate counting that may be helpful for diabetics who are also on a renal diet.

- National Renal Foundation (NKF): For those with renal disease, the NKF website (www.kidney.org) is a great resource. It includes advice on meal preparation and a section with kidney-friendly dishes. Despite not being diabetes-specific, the supplied recipes may be modified to fit a diabetic renal diet by taking into account the number of carbohydrates and portion sizes.

- Registered Dietitian/Nutritionist: Speaking with a registered dietitian/nutritionist with experience in treating diabetes and renal disease may be very helpful. They may give continuing assistance, develop food plans that are customized to each person's requirements, and offer individualized direction. They may also instruct them on how to read nutrition labels, regulate their portion sizes, and choose foods that meet both diabetes and renal diet needs.

- Online recipe repositories: Several websites provide a large selection of recipes appropriate for both diabetic and renal diets. Popular choices comprise:

- DaVita (www.davita.com/recipes): DaVita has a sizable recipe collection that is specially made for people with renal disease. Their recipes may be found and sorted according to dietary requirements, including alternatives that are suitable for people with diabetes.

- The National Kidney Foundation's Kidney Kitchen (www.kidney.org/recipes) offers a selection of kidney-friendly meals, some of which may be appropriate for those with diabetes. Finding recipes that fit with a diabetic renal diet is made simpler by the ability to search by nutritional value in recipes.